BIG ARMS

A.S.A.P.

W/O EQUIPMENT

DISCLAIMER

This is a book written by a man who has been in a cell, where dumbbells were considered a weapon, in a situation where all alpha-male traits were taboo...

But this book is not medical advice. I am not the boss of you. If it hurts don't do it.

However these advice given really will build you bigger arms given time.

SECOND DISCLAIMER

You are about to learn something that you may not already know.

There are large pits and lots of wrinkles in peoples emotions.

Don't steal all the light, don't stink of forbidden-life. Keep your mouth shut.

Show the people your splendor instead. If you feed them light they will come like moths to flame.

The tank-top texturing described in this small volume tones your lattissmus dorsi (shield) and your shoulders, but primarily your arms (guns). If you want to tone your chest do pushups, if you want stronger legs then squat.

I will teach you techniques for arms.

Your brain shapes your body. Consider how your central nervous system stretches through your entire body.

A blunt and perhaps profane example to some, that none the less proves true, are some of the 'butch' women I have met in institution. The lone lesbian warrior with a v-shaped torso and good arms. These women were shaped this way from their personalities, mostly.

Straighten your spine and you will see the difference!

You as a human can do certain exercises in order to grow, inch by inch, row by row.

It is by your will, ultimately, that you will shape your body. The instrument is secondary.

FIRST EXERCISES

First two exercises combine isometric (static) pressure with dynamic flexing. Both isometric pressure and dynamic flexing will tone muscles by themselves, but combined they offer what is perhaps the most effective toning possible by any means.

Then this info also enables you to apply the same principles to any muscle on your body.

You should do these exercises up to six times each, making sure you spend all your available power within six repetitions.

Don't just do endless repetitions, spend all you've got!

And don't hold your breath! Breathe freely.

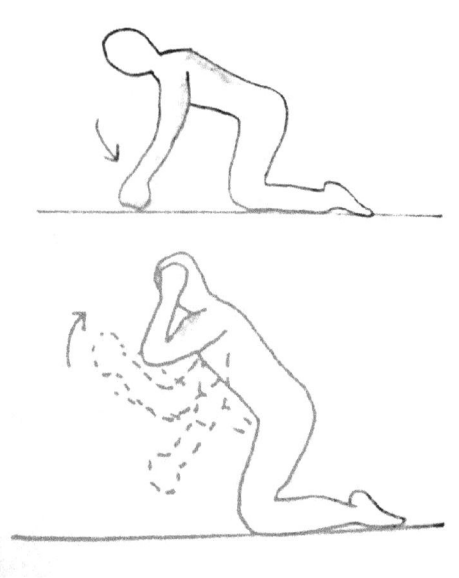

EXERCISE 1

Sit on your knees, back straight, press fists or palms down and back. Slighty bend your arms.

Feel the press in your triceps and lattissimus dorsi muscles. Like you are trying to thrust yourself forwards and up.

Then curl slowly and concentrated up and back towards yourself, tighten as hard as you can in your biceps on both arms, and slightly through the upper back.

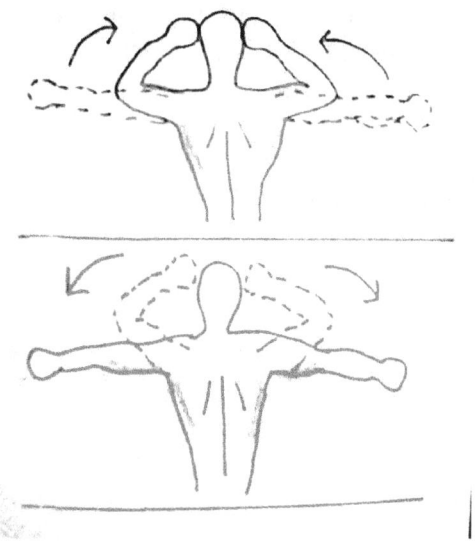

EXERCISE 2

Stand erect with your arms to the sides. Curl your arms inwards towards your head, through your biceps, until your fist or palms reach the sides of your skull. Then press static for a moment, like in exercise 1 with the hands against the floor.

Next you continue by slowly pressing the arms outwards, through your triceps, until you have extended the arms completely. This should also have secondary toning effect on your lattissimus dorsi.

These first two exercises alone can fatigue and pump your biceps/triceps very well.

You may feel charged in the hours to come, like a build-up of energy. But you may also simply get worked through and pumped. With every night there's a different moon.

*

SELF-RESISTANCE
EXERCISES

Following exercises are so called self-resistance exercises, pitting the muscles of both arms against each other. This will give you newtonic resistance precisely attuned to your actual level of strength, while at the same time respecting the natural antagonism of the upper arm. The bicep can pull, the opposing tricep can press.

Do these exercises at will, but again, don't do endless repetitions. Try to wear yourself out within six repetitions.

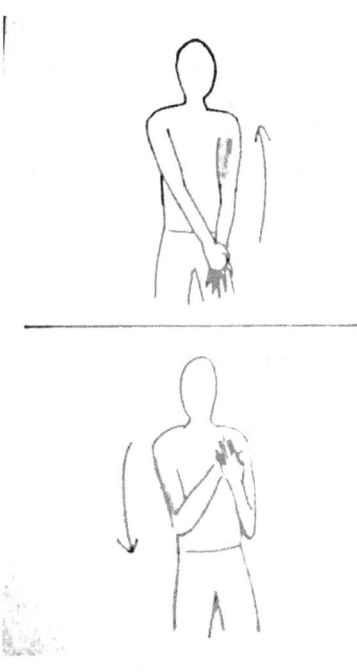

The side-curl-press shown here is perhaps even better than a seated curl to the opposite shoulder, elbow resting on the inner thigh, like a dumbbell isolation curl. But that would also be an option.

Pull as hard as you can on the curling bicep

while resisting with the opposite arm.

Then press down on the tricep of the other arm, while resisting with the first arm. Got it?

Of course you should do this with the same pull/pressure on each arm, trying to reach complete symmetry.

Don't hold your breath! But these techniques don't call for so called 'valve-breathing' either. Breathe freely.

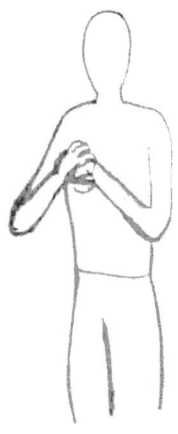

SELF-RESISTANCE
FOREARM CURL

For a complete arm-toning you really should do forearm exercises as well.

You can tone particularly your brachioradialis muscles with forearm curls.

Bend your one wrist in front of the chest, and simply try to straighten it while opposing with the other hand, like shown in the illustration.

This exercise can be done with good result, both as a static press and a dynamic motion.

And again, try to reach good symmetry on your arms.

Don't do valve-breathing, don't hold your breath. Breathe freely.

SELF-RESISTANCE
EXTENDED

You could also fold your ankles while in a seated position or lying on your back, and then flex your thighs either statically or dynamic.

To train calves perfectly you could stand in a doorway while letting your arms and shoulders act as hydraulic resistance, and then lifting your entire body through your calves.

Both these suggestions would then also hit your glutes (butt).

REACHING PROPER EFFECT

There is a bodybuilding joke that in order to get more testosterone you could watch porn to let it stimulate you, but then train your muscles instead of masturbating. Don't do this.

What you could do instead is be alone for a while, consider how the priced actress produce real tears. You will not reach tears, you will psyche yourself up! Just for a minute before training.

The love you couldn't have. The teacher that gave you wrong marks. The bitch that cheated on you. Those guys who didn't share food. Just for a minute. Then train.

When you have pulled and pressed until you really feel your heart pound, go look in a mirror. Admire your pump. Inch by inch, row by row.

*

THERAPY FOR DUDES
ONLY

There are secrets mother never told you, and father too! I can not give you the penis of a male porn-actor, but I can give you tremendous sexual function.

This is abbrievated yoga, this is not medical advice. I am not the boss of you. If it hurts, don't do it.

I will teach you how to 'lock the cock'. That is what it is called in common whore-language. Now you will be able to give the masseuse a tennis-elbow, or teach two painted ladies who's the boss.

There will be no illustrations, and women are welcome to read this as well.

You will be alone now. This time is for yourself. You should be naked, or wear loose pants. You should now sit in lotus-position with back straight, 'tailors pose'. Or you could be standing, bending forward, back straight, hands on knees.

Exhale... While inhaling through your nose contract your anus (yes you have one too), keep it contracted while moving the contraction forwards in over your scrotum (cock and balls), up into the abdominus erectus (into your navel), further up into your solar plexus... Release and relax.

This should be done as a near circular motion, all drawn through one breath in through the nose.

Your scrotum might lift slightly through the contraction. This is beneficial.

You should repeat this exercise until you really feel it, and this might happen fast.

When you have done this you should do outdoor walking or jogging, if you can get outdoors. Otherwise do something like burpees on floor. Burpees is one one the best compound calisthenic exercises.

When you train your inner muscles of the affected areas like this, you will be prone to a specific mind/body connection, allowing you to take complete control of a sexual situation as a man.

You can then 'lock the cock' and concentrate on feeling other sensations. Lust radiating through your body, your entire penis lit up like the head alone.

Be aware that something may be written between the lines.

Make it your own.

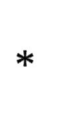